POTS: 30 DAYS TO RISE UP, POTSULAR TIPS TO HELP

Dr. Rob Wilson

POTS: 30 Days to Rise Up; Potsular Tips to Help

By Dr. Rob Wilsonn

POTS is the acronym for Postural Orthostatic Tachycardia Syndrome and as a syndrome is truly just too much to cope with. It takes on people who are often young, when the demands are excessive, and the game of life is on. It is a disorder that, despite being common, is still cloaked in bias, misunderstanding, and mystery; it is a disorder that can become all-consuming for so many reasons and in so many ways. This book is to help pause and organize, educate, reflect, and determine future goals to help navigate POTS. Potsular is a play on the word popular and helps express what has often been relevant and most noticeable throughout the journey of this condition. Take one day at a time to read, think, ponder, and plan what is and can be in your life. It takes 30 beats on a tilt table to help make the diagnosis of POTS. Now, take 30 days to help rise up from POTS.

This book is dedicated to my family and to all healthcare professionals who gave a person with POTS a chance of being believed and understood.

Contents

Day 1

Getting started is the hardest part. Here you are now, taking the first step, with some hope and possibly more doubts, together with disbelief. Is there any possibility of feeling better? Will there be better days? Will my body constantly be a reminder of how I feel? Will my brain constantly remind me of how it is *not* working? These questions will fill your awareness, but you are here now, and giving some self-acknowledgment to the fact that you are in this moment; this moment of willingness to move forward, to give something of this condition a chance. Move forward now, to give hope a chance.

Recognize in this time that as poorly as you may feel, the recognition of having this diagnosis gives you some peace of mind. The times of the unknown, uncertainty, dismissal, and fears are now a filled space since having this diagnosis of POTS – it has a name! You have a diagnosis that is present and real. This diagnosis gives you the validity that no one can remove or take away from you.

Tasks: Obtain or reclaim the reusable hydration container or bottle that you will use over and over again. Make this vessel something you would like to have around, hold, drink out of, and look at. **Goal**: will be that you will use it in 24 hours and refill it with your hydration liquid of choice. Avoid plastic disposable bottles for your health, the cost to you, and its effect on the environment. Drink 64 to 84 ounces, during the day, of your hydration of choice, whether water or some electrolyte beverage. Consume throughout the day, with a planned schedule. You will become a wellness expert in your hydration work and

1

care, a culinary Wizkid, and a good global citizen for the planet. Now that's something to aim for!

Insight: Neck pain is common in POTS. Coat hanger pain from blood not getting to the muscles in the neck, from the vertical challenge of the blood moving upward. Adrenaline can cause sympathetic muscle tightening, especially of the neck muscles. Migraines and headaches are commonly associated with POTS, which can lead to neck pain.

Day 2

You are still here, and back for more. Recognize the warrior in you to persist and be willing to keep going. There is something in you that wants more and better (recognize this and acknowledge yourself for this power).

Disappointment is the end point of failing to achieve the outcomes expected. What do we think is going to happen? What do we want to have happen? What do we want and wish from that person? Endless disappointments from family, work, school, friends, the healthcare system, and maybe even oneself are part of life with POTS.

Yes, disappointments can happen and are a reality in life, but reconfiguring and aligning expectations to be more manageable and realistic can help you on the road to wellness.

Less ideal: My medical provider, in the 15-minute appointment, could only address 2 out of 10 of my problems.

More ideal: I picked the 2 most prominent of my 10 problems, knowing my medical provider only had 15 minutes for the visit.

Less ideal: They want me to exercise 45 minutes a day. I am not an exercise person.

More ideal: This 45-minute exercise plan for a non-exerciser like me is not a good start. I will do 5-10 minutes to start with.

Task: What are the 3 biggest expectations that are not so easy for you, and that may be challenging on your road to doing better?

1.
2.
3.

What will be the mindset for you to have with these expectations, to help toward your success?

1.
2.
3.

Insight: Besides POTS impacting circulation, the adrenaline sympathetic response can alter the parasympathetic ideal of digestion. Parasympathetic is the rest and digest system. POTS patients often have many digestive issues: acid reflux, bloating, belly pain, diarrhea, constipation, food intolerance, and dry mouth.

Day 3

It is not easy feeling just sick overall. POTS patients often describe it as feeling flu-like daily. Just an overwhelming *blah* feeling blanketing one. The symptoms and experiences daily can be overwhelming. It makes sense to feel not so well overall, as the Autonomic Nervous System affects the whole body. Don't lose hope, since insights can help to give effective solutions.

Task:

What are your top 5 daily symptoms?
1.
2.
3.
4.
5

What is your most severe symptom?

The big question is whether there is a pattern or trigger for the symptom. From any of the 5 symptoms, is there a trigger or relief for the symptom? This can be food, stress, weather, activity, time of day, medicine, or a person.

What is the trigger or relief?

Insight: The body does function, in many respects, in circadian rhythms and cycles. These circadian rhythms and cycles are in the brain, heart, and kidney functions. We know that the circadian rhythms are clocks or cycles that the body will go through in sequences. Circadian rhythms and cycles influence sleep and even vital functions.

Day 4

It is in all your head! Is that familiar? Do these words haunt you? Is there a fear that these words may be thought of, spoken, or written about you? Here is a departure point for these words: it is in your head; truly, this is in your head. We are going to move it from your mind as thoughts and concepts you hold because, since the onset of your symptoms of POTS, you may have noticed triggers and factors that could make you feel better or worse. Often, in the early journey, it is the worst one you notice. It is in your head, these thoughts, the awareness, and insights. Move towards empowerment now, by having the willingness and confidence to make the association of what makes it worse and also what helps improve it. Common triggers can be foods, smells, weather, menstrual cycle, the size of a meal, and even soaps. Often these triggers and factors can be immediate or linger in their impact for a few days before they really take hold. You may find a pattern that can help improve your quality of life, as well as insights into your condition. You are also finding this confidence in yourself to claim that you can advocate for yourself for being a companion in helping yourself on your health journey. Often, being sick, especially with POTS, and with a delay in diagnosis, disbelief, and negative comments from others, your confidence is brought way down. The ability to find this pattern recognition is not just helping your health but is also a road back to confidence, obtained and reclaimed.

Task: Make a note of a bad day or days thinking about all the food you consumed, the weather, barometric pressure changes, whether a menstrual cycle occurred (sorry dudes!), quality of sleep, possible pain, and even what time of the day these occurred. You can even add more variables as triggers. Remember to define for yourself what a bad day is.

Insight: Confidence in oneself is a willingness to give oneself and one's circumstances a chance, even just a tiny, tiny, tiny, measurable chance.

Day 5

While sick, have you ever noticed the amount of stuff you collect? There is just more stuff around and, somehow, in a different way than you had before. More papers around that have words that often don't make sense. There are more plastic bottles with pills that help and often have not helped. There is often more plastic stuff from being sick. You even have certain clothing that you have now, that seems to be your sick clothes! There are, for some of you, many water bottles, compression stockings, binders, garments, massage devices, and custom-made blankets given, bought, used once, and perhaps now just lying around. This is the time, and maybe not on this day only, to declutter. Declutter to go through the process of what is helping and what is not. Does the compression gear really help or not? Declutter to physically get rid of some of these goods or maybe donate them to someone. Ask yourself, "Do I need to have twenty reusable water bottles?"

"Why am I keeping all these belongings around me?" Is the compression stocking on the floor just an expensive cat toy now? Collecting and holding on can be a necessity but could also be a window into fear, procrastination, the uncertainty of the future, organizing the present, aspects of brain fog, and perfectionism, so, to make the changes is just too overwhelming, and just too exhausting a process to simplicity. Decluttering is not just an exercise of clearing and cleaning out, but a time to think carefully and reflect. You can come to realize that something in POTS care does not work as well since not everything works after all. You may also realize you need those thirty fluffy blankets for various reasons. Maybe those blankets give you something more than warmth and comfort, like nostalgia and joy.

Task: Go through all your POTS stuff and declutter. If physically challenging, ask for help. Go through supplements and prescription medications that you do not use anymore. If a prescription needs to be eliminated in a certain manner, ask your medical provider how. Go through all of your POTS stuff with thought and reflection, to realize what is really needed and does help.

Insight: There are 10.5 units of blood volume in the human body. Our blood volume is under the influence of gravity. Our blood vessels normally respond to gravity by narrowing blood vessels to prevent blood pressure from falling.

Day 6

Having chest pain and getting it off your chest is important (excuse the pun!). Chest pain in POTS is common. You take a condition where people often have delays in diagnosis, and are labeled as crazy; the women are told in error that they are highly strung, and the men can be viewed as wimps, who look well but do not feel well. It impacts people in the prime of their lives, so there is some anger that can justifiably occur. Anger can be internalized, not always spoken of, buried, or never truly seen. Anger in POTS is not good when the hallmark of this condition is sympathetic activation of a heightened adrenaline response to keep the circulation going. This heightened adrenaline response will cause secondary offshoots in the body such as the brain experience of fight, flight, or freeze. In POTS, this fight/flight/freeze reaction becomes more readily activated. Anger is throwing kerosene onto a dumpster fire in this brain experience. Anger in POTS makes sense with the upheaval of already not feeling well; the flare-ups, waking up to just a bad day without reason, life being in chaos, and not being understood, add fuel to the fire. If we add what life may have been like before POTS that created some anger, then we have more kerosene to add to the existing fire. What is making you angry? Day 6 is dark and a challenge. You may need to stop and think and just get to know what is making you so angry. After this Day 6 exercise, you may even notice more POTS symptoms being worse since you just found some more kerosene to add to the existing fire.

Task: What is making you so angry? Do you think you can change that? Do you have someone you can talk to about these issues and problems in your daily life? Could it even be the big OK to have someone professionally to work with, to unpack and organize the anger, and to get that kerosene out of the way?

Insight: Anger has been tied to increased health risks. Are you the victim of anger?

Day 7

Fatigue: A day of rest is allowed for POTS. You have been working hard already. No shame in allowing yourself some rest. Sometimes, when being sick with this condition, one will feel shame in voicing and announcing often being tired, exhausted, worn out, not resting, needing to lie down, and feeling sleepy. Fatigue is often the daily grind of symptoms that can plague a POTS-affected person. What is fatigue as you experience it? Is it a physical, cognitive, emotional, spiritual, or more a descriptive experience of how you get through your day of limitations? Is fatigue a combination of all these states of personal being noted in the prior sentence? Is fatigue just feeling blah? Is fatigue the sense of lassitude, the state of physical and mental weariness, and lack of energy? Recognizing fatigue as part of the disorder is mandatory. Maybe not on the rest day, but thinking about what is contributing to the fatigue may be the key to your healing.

Task:

How is fatigue experienced by you?

How would you describe fatigue using different words?

What activities trigger fatigue?

What activities help relieve fatigue?

Does sleep or a nap help fatigue?

Does lying down or sitting down help fatigue?

Do you have a consistent bedtime and getting up schedule?

Do you get up often in your sleep?

Do you feel like you use too much energy to get things done?

Insight: All living things have a rest cycle.

Day 8

The jitters are part of the package deal sent to you with POTS. These jitters can be a sense of not feeling right, feeling anxious without a cause, uncertain, and with an internal or external tremor. These are all offshoots of adrenaline effects on the body, attempting to stabilize the circulation. It is part of this book's mission, to understand how this disorder can have an impact beyond circulation stabilization and neurological responses. It is also part of this book's mission, to help give the awareness and validation that these experiences are often part of the disorder. These experiences are genuine. We will explore more as to why, but for now, validation is key and mandatory. Allow yourself the needed moment to become aware that these symptoms are associated with POTS. For others, allow this to be just reinforcing that this is POTS, and perhaps for some to share with others who may have POTS. The key concept here is validation.

What has been a validating experience for you since your diagnosis of POTS?

Who has validated your diagnosis of POTS?

Insight: Validation has its origin in the Latin word, Validus, which means "strong."

Day 9

Do you awaken every morning with what feels like a hangover, but not from attending a party the night before? It is typical of POTS for you to awaken with more than the morning fog we all as humans endure and experience, but with a feeling of a hangover. This sense of having a blanket of impaired thinking, aches, pain potentially, and not sure how your body will function, is typical, especially when the condition is not stabilized or not undergoing ideal treatment. Reasons can range from poor sleep quality to quantity of sleep, medication effects, lack of medication effectiveness, and the body not moving. The body not moving can be a major contributory factor. With just lying there, the blood is not circulating in the microcirculation system, and with the impaired circulation of POTS, the necessity of sympathetic/ adrenaline compensation will lead to nighttime symptoms we see of a racing heart rate, sweating, restless sleep, and awakening. during sleep. The goal of nighttime sympathetic/adrenaline symptoms is in reaction to all the continuous POTS care of the daytime work, which will reduce the long-term need for this less-challenged nighttime microcirculation.

Task:

Is your nighttime and rest room temperature ideal for optimal rest?

Can you adjust the temperature to your body temperature needs?

Are your night clothes comfortable enough to wear and to layer on and off if needed?

When you awaken in the morning, a good tip is to hydrate well with your hydration beverage of choice of 1 to 2 liters, as soon as you awaken (though maybe urinate first).

Maybe even do about 2 to 10 minutes of simple laying-flat exercises, with just a range of motion and moving the arms and legs to get the blood moving.

Take a few minutes to read, listen to your favorite music, or revisit a quote that makes you feel good. These can help center and lift you out of the muck of what your body is telling you it is feeling.

Insight: Your body is talking to your brain all the time, and your brain is talking to your body all the time; not a message to the solution but sending messages of some affirmations of good in each direction helps in the journey.

Day 11

Belief is an odd word to use and bring to the table when some-one is sick. When you feel just nauseated, dizzy, in pain, uncertain of your body, and unpredictable, future belief seems odd and foreign. Belief has its origin in a word meaning care. It is truly interesting that to believe and have belief has some essence of care intertwined. To care about something *for you*. To believe in something *for you*. Being sick, these aspects can then be diminished and removed, by allowing time to pause to give yourself some care and faith for a moment. What and how will you give some loving care to yourself in the present and the future? What will your belief be? It could be to be less critical and less ashamed of yourself. It could be to make those medical appointments with the belief that something could become dif-ferent than in the past. There are endless options and possibili-ties of care and belief in oneself to take on this mission and ask.

Task: What will it be for you as a belief in helping you? How will you care for yourself differently?

Insight: Give yourself a chance and go for it!

Day 12

Breathing is so important. Breathing is part of life. Breath work can help in the POTS work of understanding how your body is functioning and also in its dysfunction. Breath work can also help as a tool to help the sympathetic nervous system response. When you take a deep breath inhale), your lungs inflate with air that is needed, but also reduces the amount of blood coming upward and to the heart. The inflated lungs create a barrier for the heart to receive all of its blood to pump forward and fill the body. So inflated lungs reduce the volume to the heart and then the amount pumped to the body. The heart compensates for the reduced amount of volume by speeding up the heart rate with inhalation. The converse happens with exhaling since the lungs are deflated and blood can get to the heart easily, thus there is less need for a rapid heart rate. So, with inhaling, the heart rate speeds up, and with exhaling, the heart rate slows down. By working with inspiration and expiration, one can have some influence on the heart rate and sympathetic tone. That all sounds good and easy, but the caveat is that often people in sympathetic states, like POTS, are so dysregulated that doing work to control breathing with inspiration and expiration can at first, and for a time, be odd, sickening, and not at all ideal. One can even still notice high heart rates on expiration.

Task:

Practice breathing in slowly for 3 seconds, then out slowly for 5 seconds. You can do this repeatedly throughout the day and as often as you desire.

If too sickening, then try to lie down and practice by allowing the diaphragm to drop to allow more relaxation of the diaphragm and belly.

Watch how tight the mouth, throat, and neck muscles are while breathing.

You can even practice nostril breathing with one nostril compressed. This exercise helps since nostril breathing is believed to be a more parasympathetic function.

Insight: During inhalation, the human body absorbs about 21% oxygen from the air.

Day 13

The unlucky number 13 is important for POTS, a condition that probably has always existed in humans. POTS comes from the aftermath of infections, trauma, head injury, pregnancy, EDS, autoimmune disease, and chronic illness. These ailments and insults to human bodies have always existed, for as long as we have been on this planet; however, POTS was first described during the Civil War period during which soldiers endured similar symptoms of fatigue, racing heart rate, dizziness, light-headedness in standing up, and inability to function in daily life. Not much of what soldiers experienced led to what was then called a Soldier's Heart (the heart was fine), and what we know as now as POTS. Treatments were bedrest, loose clothes, and often an antiquated medicine, called Digitalis. Moving forward, POTS has been redefined in ways similar to DaCosta Syndrome, Neurocirculatory Asthenia, Irritable Heart, and Grinch Syndrome. Most of these labels did not help except to focus on heart labeling, though the heart was fine and was only used in the over-labeling of a psychiatric cause. POTS has been an unlucky syndrome concerning lack of understanding for over a century and adding on decades more, with only recently gaining a more clinical and scientific grasp of the condition. Currently, there are no FDA-approved medicine treatments for POTS. Many approaches are based on some retrospective studies that are helpful, but not the most ideal for knowing what truly works. There are small studies that have tried interventions in exercise and other therapeutics. The issue with some studies is that they represent the POTS population at large in the study, thus showing similar benefits for all, which is not the case in reality. Is measuring the success of a study of fainting/syncope the best measure when only a small percentage of POTS sufferers faint? Would the reduction of fatigue or improvement in daily function not be better measures for success in the study? Many treatments suggested are based on what can be extrapolated to help from use in other similar autonomic disorders. POTS needs a new number besides 13.

TASK: Think about all of your daily and weekly treatments and what really helps. It is important to do this for insight. Often in the daily feeling of being sick and doing so much, one may not realize what truly helps.

Insight: Believe in your thoughts. Doubt is often an unwelcome guest!

Day 14

Blood pressure and pulse rate may not be all that one thinks they should be. Have you checked your vitals and they have been crazy high heart rate and you felt fine? Have you felt horrible and had normal blood pressure and pulse? Have you spent more time checking your heart rate and blood pressure than enjoying life? Has monitoring your vitals left you confused and not knowing what to do with the data? The body is complicated, and more is going on with POTS than just the instance of blood pressure or pulse checks. The nervous system is also involved in POTS: the nervous system responds to adrenaline and memories. Being sick often takes a toll on the body and often cannot be measured by blood pressure and pulse rate. The pain, stiffness, aches, confusion, poor sleep, and nausea, more often than not, may not be revealed by the blood pressure and pulse readings. So, the nervous system's wiring and signaling of POTS and the toll on the body of being sick, cannot be measured by taking blood pressure or pulse readings.

Task: What are your symptoms that you feel are not tied to your blood pressure or pulse being high or low? Do you have symptoms that you feel are not tied to low or high blood pressure? Do you feel you have symptoms that are not tied to a high heart rate? Please think about these symptoms: are they patterns of triggers, or patterns of relief?

Insight: There are 86 billion neurons in the human brain. These neurons form 100 trillion connections to each other. These wirings and signals are forming connections and memories of your POTS experiences and memories also, and of what it feels like to recall and experience pain, dizziness, nausea, fatigue, headaches, tingling, racing heart rate, and more. Work on POTS is often to help form new connections of these neurons in the brain.

Day 15

Yikes is a nice new word! Yikes is also being used to describe a needed pause in the new world of information content being delivered to all of us constantly; a new world of people out there of ready experts, influencers, and advisors to give ready-to-go tips, perfect remedies, and quick fixes. There are Internet quick reads and pics of must-know to give these insights. More available now are quick pics and videos of how to, bombardment of what to do, and preying on your fear, to attain their goals. Beyond this messaging of words, voices, pics, and videos, what is not revealed is how much is realistic and doable; realistic and doable for a cost of dollars, time commitments, feasibility, and true outcomes and videos telling you to eat this way and you will feel great. The videos show rapid food preparation that seems wonderful and miraculous. The videos do not show the cost of food, the preparation time, and if it will agree with your body. The videos do not go through having POTS and how it will have an impact on your health, whether you can afford the ingredients, whether the energy expenditure for food preparation is even doable for you with POTS, and will the food agree with your body having POTS. There are endless more examples and promises out there of exercises, food fixes, supplements, gadgets, and more for your POTS condition. All this stuff can also make one not feel so good about oneself. It can feel like what one is constantly not doing or just this constant negativity culture This is why Yikes is needed! Yikes is the pausing point to think of just what is realistic, feasible, and doable for oneself. "Yikes, I need to pause and think, does all this make me feel bad about myself?" Be open to Yikes for your POTS.

Task: What are the Yikes in your POTS world?

Insight: Feeling good about oneself is an active process and not just a thought

Day 16

Salty, salty! Am I that salty after all? Salt loading and ingestion are recommended and obligatory for POTS care. It becomes the automatic, default must-do for POTS care of salt loading. As we know in POTS, the great cliche that is appropriate is that one size does not fit all. Salt loading is not for all. Some people with POTS will have high blood pressure tendencies like in hyperadrenergic POTS. In this hypertension tendency, the salt loading will make blood pressure higher and perhaps the extra salt is not as ideal. Increased salt loading or salt tablets for some increase nausea, bloating, and gut dysfunction. Be mindful if salt loading or salt tablets are making your gut worse. Salt loading can make the vestibular system more challenging. The vestibular system is very salt-sensitive. Have you noticed or maybe tracked if your dizziness is better or worse by your salt load? Many people with POTS have dry mouths. Salt can burn the mouth more. Being salty can make the POTS' condition worse.

Task

How has salt helped, hindered, or worsened your POTS?

Insight: Consuming 400 milligrams of sodium, which amounts to a single gram of table salt, causes your body to retain 4 cups of water (about 2 pounds of water)

29

Day 17

The concept of "Dignity" is being introduced into sickness. This concept is paramount when sick, especially with POTS. Dignity is the sense of oneself maintaining and cultivating self-respect and pride. POTS, from the delay in diagnosis to not being believed, looking fine, but not feeling well, being dismissed as not sick, derogatory comments, and losses can challenge one and cause one to lose one's dignity. Even the topics of discussion of autonomic dysfunction, sweating, diarrhea, constipation, urine, sexual function or dysfunction, and daily activity can challenge some people's dignity. One's dignity can be altered with the need to be someone that one is not, or being more irritable, angry, wary, emotional, and present to the world, and wanting to show a side of oneself that one likes. Coveting and working on one's dignity is key when sick and must be ongoing. Showcasing the person who is and wants to be well for the world is mandatory. You are the ambassador for yourself in navigating your sickness ultimately, in actions and written and spoken word. Maintain your dignity, shine, and give respect to yourself, and leadership in professionalism as you guide yourself through your sickness.

Task

What is dignity for you while being sick?

Insight: Dignity has a Latin origin. It has origins in the meaning of "worthiness."

Day 18

Blurry is what I know! Adrenaline/sympathetic compensation to keep the blood flowing can create many other bodily responses. The primary duty of the adrenaline response is to have a high heart rate and preserve blood pressure, but there are secondary responses too. The body will have many bystander responses in thinking, digestion, skin sensations, sweating, vision, and potentially more based on what the adrenaline is trying to do as a primary duty for POTS. Many of you with POTS will have vision complaints such as blurry vision, not focusing, bright lights bothering you, glare being a challenge, and not getting your vision right in close work with devices. Many will even have these huge pupils where one will be falsely accused of using an illicit substance at times! Adrenaline response will cause pupil dilation and impaired pupil constriction; it is as if you are in danger and need to see, let light in, and be able to take it all in for protection from harm. Sounds good for true danger, but with POTS, life in the modern world causes challenges in getting through the day. Always make sure to have your eyes examined formally by a medical professional. You want your eyes examined in a medical setting. Often the issue is with this optical reaction. Working with the POTS condition can help reduce this response for many.

Task:

What other senses of hearing, skin, taste, or smell have been different since POTS? We want to recognize that the senses can be altered by POTS.

Insights:

There are 10-20 million olfactory receptor cells in humans.

The optic nerve that communicates from the eye to the brain and vice-versa has over 1 million nerve fibers in humans.

Every square inch of human skin contains 1,000 sensory nerve endings.

Day 19

If only I could take a holiday! If only my brain could take a vacation! Adrenaline and sympathetic activation will activate the brain to have you on notice that something is not right with your body in POTS. Basically, if your circulation is not working, the baroreceptor that controls blood pressure and heart rate is ultimately housed in the brain. The brain has to be notified that the body's circulation is not right. The brain has to be notified through *awareness* that the body is not right. This creates the jittery, alert, off feeling, hyper-vigilance of impending doom, and the classic fight/fright/freeze response. The brain and nervous system are all circuits that get turned on and can be ongoing. If you are in a constant adrenaline state, this brain response will be a constant potential, even if your body is okay for now. It is key to be aware that this is occurring. It is key to find ways to show your brain ways of taking off from the adrenaline experience and awareness.

This can be done medically, with medications and specific POTS care, but also with activities like wellness, gentle yoga, tai chi, music, hobbies, religion, meditation, light reading, and zoning out with a good video. Showing your brain for a few minutes or a time during a holiday or vacation how to do adrenaline reduction is needed for POTS care, often, daily, and consistently.

Task: What is your adrenaline brain?

What could your brain holiday be?

Insight: The amygdala in the brain is wired and can become activated for the fight, flight, or fright response that we can see in the adrenergic response.

Day 20

This day is about fun! A recurrent theme that I reinforce in people with chronic health disorders is that you are allowed to have fun. Yes, you often feel unwell, miserable in your body, flu-like, and have unpredictable good and bad days. Feeling sick and having fun seem mutually exclusive to each other. If one adds scrutiny of the chronically sick, especially people with POTS, the missed opportunities for fun are there. There is also an economic impact to being sick that factors into what one can do. There is the loss and exclusion of friends and family who will not accommodate or understand the disorder. There are aspects of the disorder that create obstacles and barriers of energy, pain, and bodily function to doing activities. There is scrutiny and confusion as to when a good day occurs and one with POTS can do something and then the next day cannot do the same thing. With all this, do not give up on having fun. Do not give up redefining fun with new challenges. Fun may have to be altered and different. Fun may not be on a budget now. Fun may not be all day, but a few minutes or an hour. Fun may be a new activity. Fun may be with new people, events, and surroundings. POTS people are allowed to have fun!

Task: What could be fun for you to do?

What could be simple fun for you to do?

What could be fun that you can do daily and easily?

Insight: Fun is part of the human condition.

Day 21

I have pain everywhere. It is always a shock to me when POTS patients are thought of as not having pain associated with the condition.

The following are the potential reasons (these are the common ones, and more are out there):

1. Migraines are highly common in POTS
2. Headaches are commonly associated with POTS
3. Coat hanger neck pain from low blood pressure
4. Neck spasm from adrenaline
5. Adrenaline's impact on muscles causes tightening of muscles (especially the neck, arms, back, and legs)
6. Chest pain
7. Nausea
8. Abdominal pain
9. Pelvic floor pain and pelvic floor dysfunction-associated pain
10. Small Fiber Neuropathy
11. Those who have hypermobility and Ehler-Danlos Syndrome joint disorders
12. Raynaud's
13. Skin hypersensitivity
14. Chronic pain impacts the nervous system causing central sensitization
15. Small Fiber Neuropathy
16. Burning mouth
17. Fibromyalgia
18. Restless leg
19. Muscle spasms and jerking limbs

This list is not ranked in prevalence, but according to those we see in it POTS.

Task:

What are your pain issues with POTS?

What are your best strategies for pain?

Often there are many pain issues. In a medical appointment, it can be more effective to target one or two as the goal of the visit for treatment and strategies, though many of the pain problems can intersect and overlap.

Insight: The body can remember pain. Just like a migraine can continue, pain can just be a signal at times that propagates itself. Pain can become an ongoing cycle, even once the injury is gone.

Day 22

Your body is an energy center. We need energy to get through the day. We use energy to do things. We need to take food in for energy. People with health issues, especially neurological conditions, have more taxing use of energy. If a person has a weak leg, then it takes more energy to get from point A to point B than a person without this issue. The person with a weak leg has to utilize more thought, the non-impacted leg, and the rest of the body to get to Point B. It just requires more cognitive and physical energy for that person with a weak leg to move. This is a good example of something similar in a person with POTS. That person has challenges with circulation that can tax their energy and stamina and that can make getting to Point B a challenge. If we add in aspects of the POTS pain, sleep challenges, digestion and nutritional problems, adrenaline symptoms, and social determinants, the energy usage is even higher in getting from Point A to Point B. This example of going to a designated destination really brings forth the concept of energy usage in POTS. You have to think about how to use your energy efficiently during the day. Find a good place to plan your energy usage. Energy usage for people with POTS is often the gas tank or power grid with a finite limit.

Task:

Have you noticed your energy depleted in a day?

Have you ever planned your day carefully to use your stamina and energy carefully?

Have you had some help or maneuvers to avoid overuse of energy in a day?

Have you factored in rest or help in the day or after a day of high-energy usage?

Have you ever had a POTS hangover from overdoing it? This hangover is feeling so wiped out and fatigued that one cannot function. You need to dial back then in what you do, ask for help, and see how to cut back steps in the activities.

Have you ever had an exercise hangover? This hangover can make you feel achy, fatigued, with brain fog, and not functioning. One has to dial back the effort in the exercise, as well as frequency, and time. There may need to be a rest phase before and after exercise to allow some recovery. You may need to dial back in other daily activities also to allow for the benefits of exercise for POTS.

Insight: The human body can light up a 10-watt LED bulb!

Day 23

How do I want to say it? When your body is doing this and that and more, what do you want to say about it? How do you even want to express yourself in one of those patient portal emails when you feel dizzy, weak, have brain fog, feel confused, racing heart, have headaches, are feeling off, and just feeling blah, more than what is in your baseline vocabulary perhaps? How do you even express that you are not feeling well? How do you write or speak if you are not well enough to? How do you express, "I need this" as a greater priority in a sea of symptoms of your brain and body doing odd things with POTS? It is probably key, and yes, the word is *homework* to practice how to prioritize and learn how to mentally organize one's symptoms and experiences in POTS. It may be to think about the twenty problems in how your body and brain are off in POTS. What can be the one issue in a ten-minute appointment you can address and conquer? It will not be feasible to conquer twenty issues at once, even if one feels they all must be interconnected. One has to start somewhere and take a small step forward in changing how one goes through the list, the same as organizing the experiences and symptoms. In modern medicine, there is so much information being delivered to members, including the healthcare team. The healthcare team is bombarded with too much information. Ponder, plan, and execute how to be as organized and concise as possible to deliver your problem and issue in spoken or written words. Before writing that 1000-character patient portal email, a 2-page narrative for the appointment, or a 200-page binder, take time and ponder, organize, eliminate, and think about how to be as concise as possible for your audience to have your information delivered effectively. Be an effective communicator of your healthcare needs. Read it again and hold before sending that patient portal email. Can that binder of records be trimmed down to only the needed documents such as the tilt table and your last medical appointments? Have you lost time or your audience in an appointment because of too many pages of written narrative?

Task:

What will be the one issue to work on for your next medical appointment?

Can you re-read your patient portal email and possibly think of being more concise?

Can I make my medical binder effective at only 10 to 20 pages?

Can I have a medical binder be the first tier of need-to-know medical records, and then the second tier of less need-to-know records?

Do I need to send this message on the patient email portal?

Insight:

Electronic Health Records are associated with burnout in healthcare workers; more time in front of a computer than direct patient care allowed.

Day 24

A body in motion does help. This is the darkest and most taboo of the POTS condition, to discuss the word **EXERCISE**. It is a four-letter word figuratively speaking! Exercise can be viewed as just foul for many when sick. To discuss exercise for POTS is a hard topic when one feels near to fainting, fainting, nauseated, pain, sick, and just toxic. Exercise has been studied and found to help POTS and to be beneficial.

Here are the themes of exercises, or as I said, body in motion, to help POTS

1. Strong legs help circulation.
2. After the heart, the legs are the next best circulation chamber of the body.
3. Exercise helps in controlling heart rate in the long term.
4. Exercise can help long-term with mood, pain, and rest as well.
5. Realize what you can do in exercise. Do only what you can. Go slow and low as you go. This means, for example, that for some it can be lying down for 2 to 5 minutes per day, going at a snail's pace, maybe for months. Do what you can do that makes sense for you and does not render you feeling worse afterward or the next day.
6. Work with, ideally, a POTS-literate physical therapist, exercise physiologist, personal trainer, or medical provider to find the ideal and compassionate body in motion for you.
7. Realize that the body in motion will take time of perhaps a year or longer to find benefit from. There will

be setbacks and days of having to stop. Be patient and kind to yourself during this time. Resume a lighter and simpler routine needed after a setback or after a pause in exercising.

Task:

What body in motion have you done before?

What is a feasible and realistic body in motion for you?

What will be a realistic goal for you?

What could be your obstacles and setbacks?

How can you make it fun for you?

Insight: Yoga has been around for about 5,000 years. Many people with POTS do not like yoga, with maneuvers like their heads over their shoulders but find help with restorative poses chairs, and postures to accommodate their needs.

Day 25

The body at rest stays at rest. There is so much self-care in POTS to do all day, with hydration, meals, energy planning of how to use one's body, hygiene, eating, exercising, and medical care that it can be exhausting. Sometimes it is important to be at rest and just pause. One can be doing so much every day in self-care that all day is self-care. The day and angst are consumed by a schedule of self-care. It is time to take a rest. Take pauses in the day to rest and just be. For some, this may seem to be all one does, just resting. But this is more of a deliberate rest state of taking one's body and brain to a potential calmness and showing the container of your body and brain to be a place of adrenaline reduction.

Task:

What is your best way to rest in a moment?

How can you plan to rest in the day for 5-15 minutes, without napping or sleeping?

What is your best way to get your brain and mind distracted from awareness to give it a pause and rest? How do you find the best way to give your awareness a pause from constantly not feeling well?

Insight: Your brain is still active in sleep. Sleep helps your brain clean up toxins in the brain that build up while awake.

Day 26

Too much is just too much! Often, in this diagnosis, one has to be one 's own ally to find information and data to acquire to help oneself. Time after time, not finding answers leads one to be the one to pursue answers. A person with POTS can spend countless hours searching social media and the Internet for information to help, clicking and searching for what could be the next advice and insight. Social media can be a labyrinth of endless options and confusing trappings, trappings that seem uncertain are not a help; that's for sure! Trappings that can make it seem too easy to be true. Trappings of selling goods that border on medical predatory hunting on your vulnerability. Trappings of people promoting better lives with the outcomes of their offerings. Trappings of there is no way out. Trappings of not knowing just what is true! There is information out there and there is misinformation as well. Just as there is misinformation on the news front, the healthcare world can have this sad offering too. As a person with POTS, one just wants help and correct answers with the goal of feeling better. The reality is that trappings can lead to not feeling better though. The trappings can lead to more uncertainty, worry, angst, hurt, doubt, and poor outcomes. With a diagnosis that interfaces with a population that is tech-savvy and social media-engaged, one has to be hyper-aware of these realities. The search for information needs to be deliberate, intentional, timed, planned, and reflective, and then one has to be done with it at some point!

Task:

Deliberate: What are your resources used as information to find help and answers? What is their credibility? What are they really giving you, you have to ask yourself. Are they giving you answers, community, commiseration, or validation?

Intentional: When engaging with the information, what is it you want? This builds on the deliberate aspect, but more on an awareness of oneself as to why and what you want from the searches.

Timed: How much time are you spending looking for information, or on social media/Internet? Should you restrict your time? What does your cell phone tell you of your usage weekly, especially of Internet and social media usage? Have you ever timed yourself to just perhaps 15 minutes per day or less on social media or the Internet? Have you restricted yourself to just one day per week, for 1-2 hours of healthcare homework searching?

Planned: When you are doing your information searching and engagement on social media and the Internet, what is the purpose and work to be done? Do not be aimless or random in your search. Think about what you are doing and why.

Reflective: In your time of doing all this information finding and social media/internet searching, pause to reflect on how you feel. What emotions surface of how you feel? Do you feel happy, certain, satisfied, or relieved? Or do you feel more worried, empty, hollow, confused, or sad?

Be Done with It: Plan a time to be done with the information search. Plan to be done in a set time interval with social media and the Internet. Plan an activity to replace the device time spent searching. Be done and then be done with it!

Insight: 1 in 3 Internet minutes are spent on social media. The average USA citizen spent 2 hours and 23 minutes in 2023, using social media platforms.

Day 27

It could be time to draw the line! People like to make comments about people who are sick. People like to give advice, especially to those who are sick. There will always be new people in your life to do this and there will be current people who are doing this. There will also be historical people in your life who are guilty of this. People who are sick often just accept this as a given. They just receive the comments: they welcome all the good words and often also the not-so-good ones. When you are sick, you may have re-entry into your life of historical people who were not always good to you, based on the consequences of what being sick has done to you, but you need these historical people now, to survive in daily life. You have current people with whom you may have challenging relationships, and the sickness has added more problems. There are the new people who enter while you are sick, who are there to help but often hurt you. It can be a time to think about boundaries and draw some lines, whether with your internal conversations or direct conversations and planning. Awareness that this is occurring is paramount in relationships. Often, one cannot change these relationships based on survival and necessities, but having insight is key to realizing that you are vulnerable. If you can find ways to gently plan simple boundaries concerning rules and plans of what can be said and done in these relationships, it will be a huge step forward for you. Even to just express these concepts will be easier than to make changes.

Task:

Who are these relationships with?

Can you define for those people, language that will not be used? For example, I will not use words like "try harder" or "Are you feeling lazy today." Can you set some boundaries and rules of kind language, advice restriction, time to give advice, and what type of advice or help you want to receive?

Can you share the hurt you feel with these people?

What are the vulnerabilities that render you aligned to these relationships?

Insight: In the USA, over half of adults say they have 1-3 close friends; 8% say they have no close friends.

Day 28

I am as red as a tomato but I cannot eat tomatoes at all any-more! Do you know this person? Is this person you? Many people with POTS will notice more allergies with the disorder. We may not get into the complete mast cell activation syndrome in great detail here, but POTS and allergies co-exist. The autonomic nervous system is a relationship of the interaction and partnering of the nervous, gastrointestinal, endocrine, and immune systems. Many people with POTS will notice that besides the typical POTS symptoms, new onset of food allergies, rashes, sensitivities to soaps and lotions, and medication challenges appear. Many will have a confirmed mast cell activation that shows this hyperactive, allergic response as simplistic. Labs for mast cells can be normal for these often very fastidious lab specimens to capture positive results. Mast cell activation is often a clinical diagnosis rather than a lab confirmation. Adrenaline can spike the allergy response. Gut disorders of POTS can create many food issues as noted above. High adrenaline can cause flushing. Basically, we see many allergies with POTS. Recognizing that this occurs is important and finding ways not to be submerged by daily life because of what being allergic is doing to you, is also important.

Task:

What are your allergies?

What are the best ways to maintain ideal nutrition for your allergies?

How do you cope best with your allergies?

What is your next-best future step to take to control your allergies?

Insight: The flight-fight-fright response of the sympathetic system leads to adrenaline release that can lead to immune response such as mast cell activity of histamine release.

Day 29

The gastrointestinal system is the organ system that is often impacted by POTS. Besides the POTS' influence on the micro-circulation, we see issues in the gastrointestinal system, the gut. POTS causes a high sympathetic adrenergic state. This sympathetic/adrenergic state of the classic sense of fight, flight, or freeze is the opposite of the parasympathetic/vagal of rest and digestion. One cannot rest and digest in this sympathetic/adrenergic state. We see the following symptoms at times in the POTS, antagonizing the gut's ability to digest:

1. Dry mouth
2. Tight throat and throat pain
3. Challenge to swallow
4. Acid reflux
5. Bloating
6. Nausea
7. Hiccups
8. Food sensitivities.
9. Abdominal pain
10. Diarrhea
11. Constipation
12. Diarrhea and constipation
13. Tenesmuses need to always defecate
14. Burning mouth
15. More symptoms, probably, than listed here.

Treating and being aware of the sympathetic state's impact on the gut is key to helping this part of the body.

Task: Have you noticed when your POTS is bad your gut is also bad? Try working with the POTS' adrenaline reduction to see if it helps the gut.

Insight: The origin of the word gut is tied to a reference to intestines. The gut has been viewed, since the Middle Ages, as the seat of the emotions, and the inner parts as the seat of pity or kindness.

Day 30

!!!

You are!

You are!

You are!

You are a person who, each day, does what you can for stamina, perseverance, and trying more than you know.

Moving forward, take lessons from the days you have learned, go back, read again, be willing to try new insights, believe in yourself intentionally, and see, actively, all that is good in yourself.

You are!

You are!

You are!

You are more of something achieved and more able than you know and are. You are a person of possibilities. Don't allow sickness to define you or be you. You are more and then some! Be the friend you need for yourself. This day is probably the one you need to hold onto the most going forward, to be actively kind to yourself.

Printed in Great Britain
by Amazon